THE CASTOR OIL BIBLE

UNLOCK HOLISTIC HEALTH AND ORGANIC BEAUTY—DISCOVER 50 + DIY CASTOR OIL RECIPES FOR ANTIAGING, RADIANT SKIN AND STRONG HAIR | INCLUDES EXCLUSIVE BONUSES

NANCY DAVID

Copyright © 2024 by Nancy David

TABLE OF CONTENTS

CHAPTER 1

THE SCIENCE OF CASTOR OIL

Unpacking the Science: What Makes Castor Oil Special?

Castor oil, a substance widely recognized for its remarkable health and beauty benefits, is derived from the seeds of the Ricinus communis plant. The magic behind its potency can be primarily attributed to its unique chemical composition, particularly the presence of ricinoleic acid. This singular component not only distinguishes castor oil from other plant oils but also drives most of its therapeutic properties, making it a staple in traditional and modern health and beauty regimens.

Ricinoleic acid, an omega9 fatty acid, comprises about 90% of castor oil's fatty acid content, a rarity in the botanical world. Its structure allows it to penetrate deep into the skin and the intestinal walls, which enhances its effectiveness in various topical and medicinal applications. This deep penetration is crucial for delivering nutrients directly to the body tissues that need them most, promoting better health and more effective healing processes.

The anti-inflammatory qualities of ricinoleic acid are one of its main advantages. While the body naturally responds to injury or illness with inflammation, persistent inflammation can cause a host of other health problems, including allergies, heart disease, and arthritis. By topically using castor oil, pain and inflammation can be reduced without the negative effects of synthetic drugs. This makes it an excellent natural treatment for surface level inflammation, such as acne and deeper tissue inflammation.

Additionally, ricinoleic acid acts as a humectant, which helps maintain moisture by preventing water loss through the outer layer of the skin. This moisturizing property is particularly beneficial for those with dry skin conditions, providing a natural method for enhancing skin hydration and elasticity. The result is not only healthier skin but also a more youthful appearance. Hydrated skin shows fewer signs of aging, such as fine lines and wrinkles.

Beyond skincare, the effects of ricinoleic acid extend to hair health. Its ability to lock in moisture and promote scalp health makes it an effective natural remedy for dandruff and other scalp disorders. Moreover, castor oil stimulates blood circulation to the scalp, enhancing the growth of healthier, stronger, and more lustrous hair. This circulation also means that hair follicles receive more of the nutrients necessary for healthy hair growth, further amplified by the fatty acids and vitamin E found in castor oil.

Castor oil's impact on the digestive system is another compelling aspect of its science. When consumed, ricinoleic acid exerts a mild laxative effect by promoting the movement of the muscles that push material through the intestines, helping clear the bowels. This action can be particularly beneficial for those dealing with constipation, allowing for a gentle, effective, natural method of promoting regular bowel movements.

The antibacterial properties of ricinoleic acid must be noticed. It inhibits the growth of bacteria that contribute to skin infections and acne, making castor oil a dual action remedy that hydrates the skin while protecting it from pathogens that can cause breakouts and other skin issues. For those looking for a holistic approach to skin health, this dual functionality makes castor oil a valuable addition to their skincare arsenal.

Despite its myriad benefits, it's essential to use castor oil correctly to avoid any potential side effects. While generally safe for topical application, some individuals may experience irritation, especially with undiluted use. Adverse responses can be avoided by doing a patch test prior to using castor oil. It's important to follow advised doses while using internal products because overindulging might cause diarrhea, stomach discomfort, or other digestive issues. Consult a healthcare provider before beginning any new therapy, particularly if you are pregnant or have underlying medical problems.

The unique chemical makeup of castor oil, dominated by ricinoleic acid, makes it an exceptional product for natural health and beauty treatments. From its strong moisturizing effects and anti-inflammatory properties to its ability to improve hair health and aid digestion, castor oil offers a versatile, effective solution to many common health and beauty challenges. Castor oil stands out as a material that provides a wide range of advantages validated by both historical use and contemporary scientific study, particularly as more people look for holistic and natural goods.

Investigating Side Effects: Precautions and Safe Usage

Like any natural remedy, castor oil is celebrated for its extensive range of health and beauty benefits. However, some negative effects need to be considered to guarantee safe and efficient usage. Understanding these side effects, as well as adhering to guidelines for safe usage, can help minimize any risks associated with both the topical and internal applications of castor oil.

Most people believe that topical castor oil treatment is harmless; however, some people may experience adverse responses to it. Skin rashes, itching, or swelling are possible manifestations of these responses. More severe dermatitis may occur in especially sensitive people. Therefore, before adding castor oil to your normal routine for health or beauty, you must conduct a patch test. To conduct a patch test, dab a little amount of castor oil into a skin patch within your forearm. After applying a bandage, give the region at least several hours to rest. It is generally okay to use the oil elsewhere in your body if there is no negative reaction.

Castor oil sensitivity can be lessened for people with sensitive skin by diluting it with another carrier oil, like coconut or almond oil. This dilution is especially important when using castor oil on delicate areas, such as the face or the skin around the eyes.

In addition to allergic reactions, some people might experience clogged pores or acne from the use of castor oil, particularly if it is applied in excessive amounts. Due to its thickness, castor oil may leave a barrier on the skin that, if not thoroughly cleaned off, might harbor germs or dead skin cells. Thus, it's important to use it sparingly and cleanse the skin thoroughly after its use, especially if you have acne prone or very oily skin.

The internal use of castor oil warrants more caution due to its potent laxative effects. While it can effectively relieve constipation, improper use can lead to several undesirable effects. The most common of these is diarrhea, which can occur if one ingests too much castor oil. Dehydration and electrolyte abnormalities may result from this, particularly if the diarrhea is severe or persistent. It is essential to start with a small dosage and increase it only as necessary to mitigate this risk. Adults typically should consume at most 0 milliliters at a time and should always consult a healthcare provider before using them.

Another potential side effect of consuming castor oil is abdominal pain or cramping. Since castor oil stimulates the intestines' muscles, these symptoms may be severe. Those who have irritable bowel syndrome or other digestive problems should use extreme caution and see a healthcare provider before taking castor oil to alleviate constipation.

Additionally, castor oil should not be used internally during pregnancy without medical supervision. It has been historically used to induce labor, and ingesting it can stimulate the uterus, potentially leading to premature contractions. Only a healthcare provider's advice should be sought before using castor oil for this reason.

In terms of general precautions, both topical and internal use of castor oil should always be done in moderation. Regularly consuming castor oil as a laxative over extended periods can lead to dependency, reducing the intestines' natural ability to function without the stimulus. When the use of castor oil is discontinued, this could lead to chronic constipation issues.

It's also wise to purchase cold pressed, pure, organic castor oil to avoid contaminants and additives that can cause additional health issues. Quality can significantly impact the safety and effectiveness of castor oil, whether used topically or internally.

Castor oil offers many benefits, but it also has potential drawbacks. By understanding and respecting these side effects and adhering to recommended guidelines for safe usage, users can fully enjoy the many advantages of castor oil while minimizing any risks. Always keep communication open with a healthcare provider, especially when considering new treatments or natural remedies, to make sure they are suitable for your unique lifestyle and health circumstances.

Thank You for Reading!

We appreciate you taking the time to read our book. Your feedback is incredibly valuable to us and helps us improve our future publications.

Why Your Review Matters:

Your review not only helps us understand what we did well and what we can improve but also helps other readers make informed decisions about purchasing this book. Your insights contribute to a better reading experience for everyone.

How You Can Share Your Review:

Through Amazon.com:

- Go to the Amazon page where you found my book
- Navigate to the 'Customer Reviews' section
- Click on 'Write a customer review' to share your valuable insights

Instant QR Code Access: Scan the QR code below with your smartphone to be directed to the Amazon review section

Thank you again for your support!

CHAPTER 2

SOURCING AND TYPES OF CASTOR OIL

From Plant to Product: How Castor Oil Is Made

The journey of castor oil from plant to product is a fascinating process that begins with the cultivation of castor beans and ends with the extraction of oil. This transformation not only involves meticulous steps to ensure the quality of the oil but also varies significantly based on the extraction method used. Understanding these processes offers insight into why castor oil is revered for its numerous health and beauty applications.

The Ricinus communis plant, a species of flowering plant in the Euphorbiaceae spurge family, is the source of castor beans. The plant is robust and can grow in a variety of environmental conditions. However, it thrives best in tropical and subtropical climates where there is ample sunlight and well-drained soil. The castor plant is relatively fast growing and reaches maturity when it begins to bear large, spiky seed pods. Each pod contains seeds that are the source of castor oil. These seeds are unique in appearance and have a bold, mottled pattern, but they include the potent toxin ricin, making them extremely hazardous if ingested before processing.

Harvesting castor beans is the first critical step in the production of castor oil. It typically occurs when the seed pods have dried on the plant and begin to split open, indicating that the seeds are ripe. Workers often wear protective clothing during harvest to handle the toxic seeds safely. The seeds are then collected and dried in the sun for several days to reduce their moisture content, which facilitates the extraction of the oil.

Once dried, the castor seeds undergo a cleaning process to remove dirt, debris, and any residual hulls. This is crucial as impurities can affect the quality and safety of the oil. Following cleaning, the seeds are ready for the oil extraction phase, which can be done through various methods, including cold pressing and refining.

Cold Pressing

Cold pressing is a highly regarded mechanical extraction technique that maintains the oil's inherent properties. In this process, the castor seeds are pressed through an oil press machine without the use of heat. This method ensures that the oil does not lose its nutritional properties due to high temperatures. The pressure exerted by the machine causes the seeds to release their oil, which is then collected. The resultant oil is clear, light yellow, and characterized by its purity and mild aroma. Cold pressed castor oil is highly valued for therapeutic and medicinal purposes because it retains most of the beneficial nutrients and enzymes present in the castor seeds.

Refining

In contrast to cold pressing, refining involves a series of processes that can include heating, neutralization, and bleaching, which purify the oil but can also alter its chemical structure. Refined oil is lighter in color and has less odor than coldpressed oil. The refining process begins with heating the castor seeds to a high temperature, which helps to increase the yield of oil and kills any remaining toxins. The extracted oil is then treated with a chemical solvent that helps remove impurities.

Afterward, the oil undergoes neutralization to remove free fatty acids that can contribute to its degradation. Bleaching is the next step, which improves the color of the oil by removing colored impurities. Finally, the oil may be deodorized to remove any residual odors, resulting in a much milder scent compared to cold pressed oil. Although refined castor oil is often less expensive and more visually appealing, it may need some of the nutrients found in the unrefined version.

Both cold pressing and refining have their places in the castor oil market. Cold pressed castor oil is preferred for its health benefits and is often used in the food, medicine, and skin care industries. Meanwhile, refined castor oil is commonly used in cosmetics and industrial applications where the oil's appearance and odor may be factors, and the nutritional content is less of a concern.

The process from plant to product for castor oil is intricate and requires careful handling to ensure the highest quality oil is produced. Whether cold pressed or refined, each method offers different advantages that make castor oil a versatile and valuable commodity in various industries. By understanding these processes, consumers can make informed choices about the type of castor oil that best suits their needs, whether for health, beauty, or industrial purposes.

Cold Pressed vs Refined: Which Type Should You Use?

When deciding between cold pressed and refined castor oil, understanding their different benefits and drawbacks is crucial to determine which type suits various needs, from therapeutic applications to beauty treatments and industrial uses.

Cold pressed castor oil is produced by pressing the castor seeds without heat, preserving most of the oil's natural properties. This method keeps essential nutrients and enzymes intact, making cold pressed oil highly valued for its quality and effectiveness. It is rich in nutrients due to the absence of heat and chemicals in processing, offering significant benefits for skin and hair health through its moisturizing and anti-inflammatory properties. Additionally, because it is processed without chemicals, it remains pure and safe, especially for sensitive skin and internal consumption. The oil also retains a better taste and a more pleasant aroma than its refined counterpart.

However, there are some limitations. Cold pressed castor oil typically has a shorter shelf life because natural impurities are not removed during processing. It is also more expensive because the cold pressing process yields less oil compared to other methods. Its high viscosity and strong odor can make it less suitable for certain industrial applications where these factors are a concern.

Cold pressed castor oil is especially ideal for medicinal purposes and beauty applications, such as skin moisturizers and hair conditioners, where the preservation of nutrients is crucial for maximum effectiveness.

On the other hand, refined castor oil undergoes processes that include heating, neutralizing, and sometimes bleaching and deodorizing, extending its shelf life and improving its color and odor, making it more appealing for cosmetic and industrial purposes. The refining process produces an oil with a neutral odor and taste, which is preferred in cosmetic products like lipsticks and creams, and results in a clearer, more transparent oil that is suitable for products where a neutral appearance is desired. The removal of impurities also means refined castor oil has a longer shelf life, making it stable for long-term storage.

The drawbacks of refined castor oil include the potential loss of nutrients, such as ricinoleic acid, due to the high temperatures and chemicals used in refining. These processes can degrade many of the oil's beneficial properties. Additionally, the use of chemical solvents in some refining processes might leave residual chemicals in the oil, which could be a concern for individuals with sensitive skin or allergies.

Refined castor oil is often used in industrial applications where lubricating properties are essential, such as in the manufacture of plastics and paints. It is also commonly used in mainstream cosmetics, where an odorless, colorless oil is necessary.

The decision between cold pressed and refined castor oil depends on the intended use of the oil. Cold pressed castor oil is the preferable choice for applications requiring maximum health benefits, particularly for direct application to skin or hair. However, refined castor oil is more suitable for industrial uses or cosmetic applications where odorless and colorless oil is required.

By understanding these details, consumers can select the type of castor oil that best meets their specific needs, ensuring they harness the appropriate benefits for their health, beauty, or industrial purposes. Whether for personal care or professional use, the right kind of castor oil can provide the necessary advantages for each unique application

Organic Castor Oil: Why It Matters

Organic castor oil is a high-end choice for anyone searching for the best oil available for use in wellness, cosmetics, and health applications. 'Organic' oil is designated as such because it was produced in compliance with strict regulations designed to protect the environment and guarantee that no hazardous chemicals were used in the finished product. Understanding the advantages of using organic castor oil, along with the certification processes and the impact of organic farming practices, can provide valuable insight into why this type of oil is often considered superior to nonorganic alternatives.

The primary advantage of organic castor oil lies in its purity and quality. Since synthetic fertilizers and pesticides are prohibited under organic agricultural techniques, the castor beans used to make the oil are cultivated without the use of hazardous chemicals. This minimizes the risk of contaminants that could compromise the oil's quality and safety, making organic castor oil a safer choice, especially for use in skincare and therapeutic applications.

Furthermore, organic castor oil is often richer in nutrients compared to nonorganic varieties. Soil management practices in organic farming aim to enhance soil fertility naturally, leading to more robust plant growth and, consequently, seeds that are higher in nutritional value. This produces an oil that is devoid of artificial chemicals and has a greater concentration of healthy substances like ricinoleic acid and antioxidants. These compounds are crucial for the oil's anti-inflammatory and moisturizing properties, making organic castor oil particularly effective for healing, hydrating, and nourishing the skin and hair.

Another significant advantage of using organic castor oil is its environmental impact. Organic farming techniques foster ecological balance and biodiversity, maintaining the health of farming environments. By avoiding synthetic chemicals, organic farming reduces pollution and soil degradation, preserves water quality, and supports wildlife. Choosing organic castor oil supports these ecofriendly initiatives and is consistent with the ideals of customers who place a high value on ethical production processes and sustainability.

Organic product certification is a laborious procedure that guarantees the products fulfill stringent national and international criteria. In the United States, for instance, organic products must comply with the standards set by the United States Department of Agriculture (USDA). The castor beans must be produced on land that has been free of banned contaminants for at least three years prior to harvest in order for the castor oil to receive organic certification. Moreover, farming practices should foster resource cycling, promote ecological balance, and conserve biodiversity. This certification is not only a mark of quality but also reassures consumers about the product's compliance with environmental and health standards.

Organic cultivation methods significantly impact the potency and purity of castor oil. These methods strongly emphasize using organic fertilizers, such as compost and green manure, that enhance the structure and health of the soil. Healthier soil produces healthier plants, which in turn yield seeds with higher nutritional content. Additionally, the absence of synthetic pesticides means the oil is less likely to contain pesticide residues that could trigger allergic reactions or other health issues.

Moreover, the biodiversity encouraged by organic farming practices leads to more resilient agricultural systems. In addition to lowering the need for chemical treatments and further guaranteeing the purity of the castor oil produced, diverse ecosystems are more adapted to control illnesses and pests.

Organic castor oil offers numerous benefits over nonorganic alternatives, including higher quality, the absence of harmful chemicals, enhanced nutritional content, and a positive environmental impact. The stringent certification processes that organic products undergo add an extra layer of assurance for consumers, making organic castor oil the preferred choice for those committed to health, sustainability, and environmental stewardship. Whether used for personal care, health remedies, or other applications, organic castor oil provides a pure, potent, and ethically produced alternative that aligns with the needs and values of health-conscious consumers.

CHAPTER 3
CASTOR OIL FOR SKIN CARE

Introduction to Natural Skin Care with Castor Oil

Ricinus communis seeds are the source of castor oil, which is useful in any natural skincare routine because of its exceptional moisturizing and cleaning qualities. Its versatility and effectiveness stem from its unique chemical composition, particularly its high content of ricinoleic acid, which provides profound benefits for skin health. This natural oil can be integrated seamlessly into daily skincare practices to enhance skin hydration, cleanliness, and overall health.

Castor oil's hydrating properties are primarily due to its rich content of fatty acids, especially ricinoleic acid. This unique fatty acid helps to lock moisture into the skin by preventing water loss through the skin's outer layer. It draws moisture from the air into the skin by acting as a natural humectant, which is especially advantageous for those with dry or flaky skin. Frequent use of castor oil can improve the elasticity and young shine of the skin by making it softer, smoother, and more malleable.

The application of castor oil for hydration is straightforward and can be adjusted to suit different skin types. For direct application, a few drops of castor oil can be warmed between the hands and gently massaged into the skin, focusing on dry areas. This method is especially effective when done in the evening, allowing the oil to penetrate deeply and work its magic overnight. For those with oily skin, mixing castor oil with lighter oils like jojoba or grapeseed oil can create a balanced moisturizer that hydrates without leaving an overly greasy residue.

In addition to its moisturizing benefits, castor oil is also a potent cleanser. Its thick consistency helps lift away dirt and impurities from the skin's surface, making it an excellent choice for a natural cleanser. Furthermore, the oil's antibacterial properties help to keep the skin clean and reduce the prevalence of acne causing bacteria. This dual action of cleansing and offering antibacterial protection makes castor oil an effective component in managing acne prone skin.

A popular method of utilizing castor oil's cleansing properties is the oil cleansing method. This involves applying castor oil directly to dry skin and massaging it to help dissolve impurities and makeup. After massaging, a warm, damp washcloth can be placed over the face to open the pores, allowing the oil to carry away dirt and toxins. The washcloth can then be used to gently wipe away the oil, leaving the skin clean and hydrated.

Integrating castor oil into a daily skincare routine can be done in several effective ways. For morning routines, castor oil can be used as a gentle cleanser before applying makeup. To make sure the skin stays moisturized all day, a tiny bit of oil can be rubbed into the skin and then removed with a warm towel. A light moisturizer can follow this.

Castor oil can play a more intensive role in the evening. It can be used as part of a double cleansing routine, where the oil is first used to remove makeup and impurities, followed by a water-based cleanser to ensure all traces of dirt are removed. After cleansing, applying a thin layer of castor oil as a night moisturizer can help repair and rejuvenate the skin overnight. Its deep moisturizing properties are particularly beneficial during the night when the skin's repair processes are most active.

Beyond daily routines, castor oil can be used in special treatments to tackle specific skin concerns. For instance, you may make a castor oil pack by soaking a piece of cloth in the substance and applying it to your skin while it's heated to a comfortable temperature. This treatment can soothe inflamed skin, reduce redness, and accelerate the healing of skin conditions such as eczema or psoriasis.

Additionally, castor oil can be combined with other natural ingredients to create masks and scrubs tailored to specific skin needs. Mixing castor oil with turmeric and honey can produce a powerful anti-inflammatory and moisturizing face mask, ideal for soothing irritated skin and brightening the complexion.

Castor oil offers a versatile and effective solution for various skin care needs, from deep hydration to thorough cleansing. Its natural properties make it suitable for integration into daily skincare routines, providing a simple yet profound way to maintain healthy, radiant skin. By leveraging the unique benefits of castor oil, individuals can enjoy a more natural approach to skincare that nurtures and protects the skin holistically.

Scientific Studies about castor oil for Skin Care

Castor oil has been the subject of extensive scientific study for its potential benefits in skincare, particularly due to its anti-inflammatory and antimicrobial properties. This body of research supports the traditional uses of castor oil, confirming its effectiveness in treating various skin conditions and enhancing overall skin health

Due in significant part to its high ricinoleic acid content, castor oil has anti-inflammatory properties that make it one of its main advantages. Ricinoleic acid has been shown to have strong anti-inflammatory properties by research published in the International Journal of

Inflammation. These benefits may prove helpful in the treatment of psoriasis and eczema. The study demonstrated that when castor oil was applied to inflamed skin, it significantly reduced inflammation and discomfort. This property makes castor oil an effective natural remedy for reducing swelling, redness, and pain associated with inflammatory skin conditions.

An additional study published in the Journal of Medicinal Food indicates that topical castor oil treatment can improve tissue inflammatory repair. This study shows that by promoting the creation of lymphocytes, which are essential for the immunological response, castor oil not only lowers inflammation but also quickens the healing process. This ability to promote faster healing makes castor oil particularly useful for recovering from acne outbreaks, as it helps to reduce inflammation while preventing further infections.

Castor oil's benefits for inflammation and infection are widely recognized. A pivotal study in the Journal of Clinical Microbiology revealed that it possesses potent antibacterial properties, particularly against Staphylococcus aureus, a common bacterium that can cause skin infections. The study highlighted that castor oil could inhibit the growth of these bacteria, suggesting a protective role in preventing skin infections.

Moreover, castor oil has been studied for its antifungal properties. Research published in the Journal of Ethnopharmacology explored the effectiveness of castor oil against Candida albicans, a yeast that can cause fungal infections on the skin. The findings indicated that castor oil could inhibit the growth of Candida cells, reducing the risk and severity of fungal skin infections. This antifungal activity further supports the use of castor oil in treating and preventing conditions like athlete's foot and ringworm, as well as dandruff, which can sometimes be caused by yeast overgrowth on the scalp.

Beyond its anti-inflammatory antimicrobial effects, castor oil is also recognized for its hydrating properties, which complement its therapeutic uses. Its ability to retain moisture helps keep the skin hydrated, which is essential for maintaining the skin's barrier function and overall health. This hydration is particularly beneficial in managing dry skin conditions, which can exacerbate inflammation and susceptibility to infection.

The comprehensive benefits of castor oil, as demonstrated through various scientific studies, underline its effectiveness as a multifunctional ingredient in skincare. Its ability to address inflammation, combat microbial infections, and promote hydration makes it a valuable component of both therapeutic and daily skincare routines. By incorporating castor oil into skincare products or routines, individuals can leverage these scientifically backed benefits to maintain and enhance skin health naturally.

Scientific studies have shown that castor oil has strong anti-inflammatory and antibacterial qualities, making it a great natural remedy for a variety of skin conditions. These studies provide a strong foundation for the continued use of castor oil in dermatological treatments and daily skincare, helping individuals achieve healthier, more resilient skin.

20 DIY Castor Oil Recipes for Every Skin Type

Basic Castor Oil Moisturizer- Suitable for all skin types

Ingredients:

- 2 tablespoons castor oil.
- 2 tablespoons sweet almond oil (substitute with jojoba oil for oily skin).
- 2 tablespoons coconut oil (use fractionated coconut oil for a lighter texture).
- Optional:5 10 drops of essential oil (lavender for sensitive skin, tea tree for acne prone skin, or rosehip for aging skin).

Instructions:

1. Gently melt the coconut oil in a small saucepan or double boiler over low heat.
2. Once the coconut oil is melted, remove from heat and add the castor oil and sweet almond oil Stir thoroughly to ensure all ingredients are well combined.
3. If desired, add essential oils according to your skin type needs This step is optional but enhances the moisturizer's benefits and adds a pleasant scent.
4. Allow the mixture to cool slightly before transferring it to a small glass jar Let it solidify at room temperature or place in the refrigerator for faster setting.
5. Apply a small amount to the face after cleansing, massaging gently in circular motions Allow the oils to absorb into the skin.

Nutritional Values (per serving):

- Ricinoleic Acid: Essential for hydrating the skin and reducing inflammation.
- Vitamin E: Antioxidant properties that protect skin cells.
- Lauric Acid: Provides antimicrobial and anti-inflammatory benefits.

Castor Oil and Almond Cleanser - Ideal for oily/combination skin

Ingredients:

- 2 tablespoons castor oil.
- 2 tablespoons sweet almond oil.
- Optional: 510 drops of tea tree essential oil.

Instructions:

1. In a small mixing bowl, combine the castor oil and sweet almond oil These oils blend to create a base that effectively dissolves excess sebum while maintaining skin hydration.
2. If desired, add tea tree essential oil to the oil blend Tea tree oil is known for its antimicrobial and anti-inflammatory properties, making it an excellent addition for oily and acne prone skin.
3. Mix the oils thoroughly to ensure they are well combined.
4. Transfer the oil mixture to a clean glass bottle with a secure lid for easy application.
5. To use, apply a small amount of the cleanser to a dry face Massage gently in circular motions over the entire face to lift and dissolve impurities and excess oils.
6. Wet a soft washcloth with warm water and place it over the face for a minute to open pores and enhance the cleansing effect.

7. Wipe away the oil gently with the warm washcloth, rinsing the cloth as needed Finish by rinsing your face with cool water to close the pores.

Nutritional Values (per serving):

- Ricinoleic Acid: Essential for balancing skin hydration and reducing inflammation.
- Vitamin E: Provides antioxidant protection that helps maintain skin health.

Anti-Aging Castor Serum - Perfect for aging skin

Ingredients:

- 2 tablespoons castor oil.
- 2 tablespoons argan oil.
- 1 tablespoon rosehip oil.
- Optional: 5 drops of frankincense essential oil.

Instructions:

1. In a small mixing bowl, combine the castor oil, argan oil, and rosehip oil These oils are known for their antiaging properties, providing deep nourishment and improving skin elasticity.
2. If desired, add frankincense essential oil to the mixture Frankincense is revered for its ability to reduce the appearance of fine lines, wrinkles, and blemishes, and to promote the regeneration of healthy skin cells.
3. Stir the oils together thoroughly to ensure they are well blended.
4. Pour the serum mixture into a dark glass dropper bottle to protect the oils from light, which can degrade their quality.
5. To use, apply a few drops of the serum to your face and neck after cleansing,

preferably at night Gently massage the serum into your skin using upward strokes until it is fully absorbed.

Nutritional Values (per serving):

- Ricinoleic Acid: Helps to lock in moisture and promote skin elasticity.
- Vitamin E and Fatty Acids: Present in argan and rosehip oils, these compounds support skin hydration, repair, and cell regeneration.

Castor Oil Spot Treatment - For Acne Prone Skin

Ingredients:

- 1 tablespoon castor oil.
- 1 tablespoon witch hazel.
- 2 drops tea tree oil.
- 2 drops lavender oil.

Instructions:

1. In a small container, mix the castor oil with witch hazel Castor oil is known for its anti-inflammatory properties, while witch hazel serves as an astringent to cleanse and soothe irritated skin.
2. Add tea tree oil and lavender oil to the mixture Tea tree oil is renowned for its antibacterial properties, which help combat acne causing bacteria, and lavender oil promotes healing and reduces scarring.
3. Shake the container gently to ensure all ingredients are well blended
4. To use, apply a small amount of the mixture directly onto acne spots using a clean cotton swab Use at night after cleansing and before moisturizing.

5. Let the treatment sit overnight and rinse off in the morning Repeat nightly as needed.

Nutritional Values (per serving):

- Ricinoleic Acid: Anti-inflammatory and antibacterial, helps reduce acne and skin inflammation.
- Tannins: Witch hazel's natural astringent properties help tighten pores and calm skin.

Hydrating Castor Night Cream - Best for Dry Skin

Ingredients:

- 2 tablespoons castor oil.
- 2 tablespoons shea butter.
- 1 tablespoon aloe vera gel.
- 1 teaspoon vitamin E oil.

Instructions:

1. In a double boiler, gently melt the shea butter until it's completely liquid.
2. Remove from heat and mix in the castor oil and vitamin E oil Both oils are excellent for deep hydration and adding a protective layer to retain moisture in the skin.
3. Add the aloe vera gel to the mixture and stir until the ingredients are fully combined and the texture is creamy.
4. Transfer the cream to a clean jar with a lid and allow it to cool and set at room temperature.
5. To use, apply a small amount of the cream to your face and neck in the evening after cleansing Massage gently in upward circles until fully absorbed.

Nutritional Values (per serving):

- Ricinoleic Acid: Helps to lock in moisture and reduce skin dryness.
- Vitamin E: Antioxidant properties protect the skin

from environmental stressors and aid in skin repair.

Soothing Castor and Aloe Vera Mask - Great for Sensitive Skin

Ingredients:

- 1 tablespoon castor oil.
- 2 tablespoons aloe vera gel.
- 1teaspoon honey (optional for additional moisturizing and antibacterial properties)

Instructions:

1. In a small bowl, combine the castor oil and aloe vera gel These ingredients are known for their soothing and healing properties, making them ideal for sensitive skin.
2. If desired, add honey to the mixture for its moisturizing and antibacterial benefits, which can enhance the skin's softness and clarity.
3. Mix all the ingredients until you achieve a smooth, consistent paste.
4. Apply the mask evenly over your clean face, avoiding the eye area.
5. Leave the mask on for about 0 minutes to allow the ingredients to soothe and hydrate the skin.
6. Rinse off with lukewarm water and pat your skin dry with a soft towel.
7. Follow up with a gentle moisturizer to lock in hydration.

Nutritional Values (per serving):

- Ricinoleic Acid: Provides anti-inflammatory and hydrating properties.
- Aloe Vera: Rich in vitamins and minerals, soothes and heals the skin.
- Honey: Natural humectant that draws moisture into the skin and has antibacterial properties.

Brightening Castor and Lemon Mask - Enhances Dull Skin

Ingredients:

- 1 tablespoon castor oil.
- 1 tablespoon fresh lemon juice.
- 1 teaspoon natural yogurt (acts as a gentle exfoliant and moisturizer).

Instructions:

1. In a clean mixing bowl, blend the castor oil, lemon juice, and natural yogurt until the mixture is smooth.
2. Cleanse your face thoroughly before applying the mask to ensure maximum absorption.
3. Apply the mask evenly over your face, avoiding the sensitive areas around the eyes and mouth.
4. Leave the mask on for about 10-15 minutes, as lemon juice can be potent and should not be left on the skin too long.
5. Rinse the mask off with cool water and gently pat your face dry
6. Apply a light moisturizer to soothe the skin and prevent dryness.

Nutritional Values (per serving):

- Ricinoleic Acid: Moisturizes and promotes skin health.
- Vitamin C: Found in lemon juice, helps brighten and even out skin tone.
- Lactic Acid: Present in yogurt, gently exfoliates and refreshes the skin.

Castor Oil and Clay Deep Cleansing Mask - Targets Impurities in Oily Skin

Ingredients:

- 1 tablespoon castor oil.
- 2 tablespoons bentonite clay.
- Water (enough to form a paste).
- Optional: 2 drops of peppermint oil for a refreshing feel and antibacterial properties.

Instructions:

1. In a nonmetallic bowl, mix the bentonite clay and castor oil Bentonite clay is highly absorbent and effective at pulling impurities and excess oils from the skin.
2. Gradually add water to the mixture, stirring continuously until a smooth paste is formed.
3. For an added refreshing sensation and antibacterial effect, incorporate the optional peppermint oil into the paste.
4. Apply the mask evenly to a cleansed face, avoiding the eyes and lips.
5. Allow the mask to dry for about 10-15 minutes. As it dries, the clay will help draw out impurities from the pores
6. Rinse off the mask with warm water, using gentle circular motions to exfoliate any dead skin cells.
7. Finish by patting your face dry and applying a light moisturizer to soothe the skin.

Nutritional Values (per serving):

- Ricinoleic Acid: Provides deep cleansing and helps to remove oils and impurities.

- Bentonite Clay: Rich in minerals, absorbs excess oil and detoxifies the skin.

Nourishing Castor and Avocado Facial - Deep Hydration for Dry Areas

Ingredients:

- 1 tablespoon castor oil.
- 1 ripe avocado, mashed.
- 1 tablespoon honey (optional for extra moisturization and antibacterial properties).

Instructions:

1. In a bowl, combine the mashed avocado and castor oil until well blended Avocado is rich in fatty acids and vitamins that nourish and hydrate the skin.
2. If desired, add honey to the mixture for its additional moisturizing and soothing benefits.
3. Apply the mixture to your clean face, focusing particularly on dry areas that require more hydration.
4. Leave the facial on for about 20 minutes to allow the ingredients to deeply moisturize and repair the skin.
5. Rinse the mask off with lukewarm water and gently pat your skin dry.
6. Follow up with your regular moisturizer to lock in the hydration.

Nutritional Values (per serving):

- Ricinoleic Acid: Helps to lock in moisture and reduce skin dryness.
- Avocado Oil: High in oleic acid and monounsaturated fats, making it ideal for hydrating and softening the skin.

Castor Oil Exfoliating Scrub - Removes Dead Skin Cells Gently

Ingredients:

- 2 tablespoons castor oil.
- 2 tablespoons fine sugar.
- 1 tablespoon oatmeal (finely ground).
- Optional: 2 drops of lavender essential oil for soothing properties.

Instructions:

1. Combine the castor oil, fine sugar, and finely ground oatmeal in a bowl The sugar and oatmeal serve as gentle exfoliants that won't damage the skin.
2. If desired, add lavender essential oil for its calming and soothing effects, which can be beneficial during exfoliation.
3. Mix all ingredients together until a consistent paste is formed.
4. Apply the scrub to a damp face in gentle circular motions, focusing on areas with rough or dry skin.
5. Massage gently for 2-3 minutes to allow the exfoliating ingredients to remove dead skin cells effectively.
6. Rinse off with warm water and pat the skin dry with a soft towel.
7. Follow up with a moisturizer to keep the skin hydrated after exfoliation.

Nutritional Values (per serving):

- Ricinoleic Acid: Provides hydration while removing impurities.
- Oatmeal: Offers gentle exfoliation, soothing properties, and helps absorb excess oil.

Anti-Inflammatory Castor and Turmeric Blend - Soothes and Reduces Redness

Ingredients:

- 2 tablespoons castor oil.
- 1 teaspoon turmeric powder.
- 1 tablespoon aloe vera gel.
- Optional: 2 drops of chamomile essential oil for enhanced calming effects.

Instructions:

1. In a small bowl, mix the castor oil with turmeric powder and aloe vera gel Turmeric is known for its powerful anti-inflammatory properties, while aloe vera gel provides a cooling and soothing effect.
2. Optionally, add chamomile essential oil to the mixture for its additional soothing and anti-inflammatory benefits.
3. Stir all ingredients until well combined into a smooth paste.
4. Apply the blend to clean skin, focusing particularly on areas that are prone to redness or inflammation.
5. Leave the mask on for about 15-20 minutes, allowing the ingredients to soothe and reduce redness.
6. Rinse off with cool water and gently dry the skin with a soft towel.
7. Apply a gentle moisturizer to soothe the skin further and lock in the benefits of the mask.

Nutritional Values (per serving):

- Ricinoleic Acid: Helps to soothe and hydrate the skin.
- Curcumin: Active component in turmeric, known for its anti-inflammatory and antioxidant properties.

Castor Oil Under Eye Serum Minimizes Dark Circles and Puffiness

Ingredients:

- 1 tablespoon castor oil.
- 1tablespoon almond oil.
- Optional: 2 drops of vitamin E oil for added antioxidant benefits.

Instructions:

1. In a small container, mix the castor oil with almond oil These oils are known for their gentle and nourishing properties, which are particularly beneficial for the delicate undereye area.
2. If desired, add vitamin E oil to the mixture Vitamin E is an antioxidant that helps to combat oxidative stress and rejuvenate the skin.
3. Blend all ingredients thoroughly to ensure a uniform mixture.
4. Transfer the serum into a clean glass bottle with a dropper for easy application.
5. To use, gently apply a few drops of the serum under the eyes using your ring finger, tapping lightly until absorbed Avoid pulling or rubbing the skin.
6. Apply nightly before bed to allow the oils to work overnight, reducing dark circles and puffiness.

Nutritional Values (per serving):

- Ricinoleic Acid: Helps to lock in moisture and promote skin elasticity.
- Vitamin E: Provides antioxidant protection that helps maintain skin health.

Balancing Castor Toner Restores pH Balance for Combination Skin

Ingredients:

- 1 tablespoon castor oil.
- 1 tablespoon witch hazel.
- 1cup distilled water.
- Optional: 2 drops of rosewater for additional soothing and toning properties.

Instructions:

1. Mix the castor oil with witch hazel and distilled water in a bowl Witch-hazel acts as a natural astringent, helping to tone and balance the skin without over drying.
2. If desired, add rosewater to the mixture for its soothing and hydrating effects, which are especially beneficial for combination skin.
3. Stir all components thoroughly until well combined.
4. Pour the toner into a clean bottle with a tightfitting lid or a spray top for easy application.
5. To use, apply the toner to a cotton pad and gently wipe over cleansed skin, focusing on the T-zone and any oily areas Avoid the eye area.
6. Use morning and night after cleansing to maintain optimal pH balance and prepare the skin for moisturizing.

Nutritional Values (per serving):

- Ricinoleic Acid: Helps balance oil production and reduce inflammation.
- Tannins: Witch hazel provides natural astringent properties that help tighten pores and remove excess oil.

Castor and Tea Tree Oil Acne Gel - Fights Acne Effectively

Ingredients:

- 1 tablespoon castor oil.
- 1tablespoon aloe vera gel.
- 34 drops of tea tree oil.

Instructions:

1. In a small mixing bowl, combine the castor oil and aloe vera gel Castor oil is known for its anti-inflammatory and antibacterial properties, while aloe vera gel provides a soothing and hydrating base.
2. Add tea tree oil to the mixture Tea tree oil is highly regarded for its potent antibacterial and anti-inflammatory properties, making it particularly effective against acne.
3. Stir all the ingredients until they are well combined and the consistency is smooth.
4. Transfer the gel to a clean container with a lid or a pump dispenser for easy application.
5. To use, apply a small amount of the gel directly to clean skin on affected areas Use in the morning and at night after cleansing but before moisturizing.

Nutritional Values (per serving):

- Ricinoleic Acid: Known for its anti-inflammatory and antimicrobial properties.
- Terpinenol: Active ingredient in tea tree oil, known for combating pathogens that cause acne.

Castor and Honey Healing Mask- Repairs and Calms Damaged Skin

Ingredients:

- 2 tablespoons castor oil.
- 2 tablespoons raw honey.
- Optional: 1 teaspoon lemon juice for added brightening effects.

Instructions:

1. In a clean bowl, blend the castor oil and raw honey until thoroughly combined Castor oil helps to promote healing and reduce inflammation, while honey is a natural antibacterial and humectant.
2. If desired, add lemon juice to enhance the mask's skin brightening properties Ensure to use freshly squeezed lemon juice to avoid skin irritation.
3. Mix all ingredients well to form a smooth, consistent paste.
4. Apply the mask evenly over cleansed facial skin, avoiding the eye area
5. Leave the mask on for 15-20 minutes, allowing the ingredients to deeply nourish and repair the skin.
6. Rinse off with warm water, and gently pat your face dry with a soft towel.
7. Follow up with a light moisturizer to seal in the benefits.

Nutritional Values (per serving):

- Ricinoleic Acid: Helps soothe and reduce inflammation in the skin.
- Enzymes in Honey: Aid in the natural exfoliation process and have antibacterial properties.

Rejuvenating Castor Night Oil Blend - For a Youthful Glow

Ingredients:

- 2 tablespoons castor oil.
- 1 tablespoon jojoba oil.
- 1 tablespoon rosehip oil.

- Optional: 3/4 drops of frankincense essential oil for additional antiaging benefits.

Instructions:

1. In a small mixing bowl, combine castor oil, jojoba oil, and rosehip oil These oils are excellent for skin regeneration and hydration.
2. Add frankincense essential oil if desired Frankincense is known for its powerful antiaging and skin rejuvenation properties.
3. Stir all the ingredients together until they are well blended.
4. Transfer the oil blend into a clean glass bottle with a dropper for easy application.
5. To use, apply a few drops of the oil blend to your face and neck at night after cleansing Gently massage in upward motions until the oil is absorbed.
6. Use regularly for best results, allowing the natural ingredients to nourish and rejuvenate the skin overnight.

Nutritional Values (per serving):

- Ricinoleic Acid: Promotes hydration and supports skin elasticity.
- Essential Fatty Acids: Found in jojoba and rosehip oils, crucial for repairing and regenerating skin tissues.

Protective Castor and Shea Butter Balm Shields Skin from Environmental Damage

Ingredients:

- 2 tablespoons castor oil.
- 2tablespoons shea butter.
- 1 tablespoon beeswax.

- Optional: 2 drops of lavender essential oil for soothing properties.

Instructions:

1. In a double boiler, melt the shea butter and beeswax together until completely liquid.
2. Remove from heat and stir in the castor oil, mixing thoroughly to ensure all ingredients are well combined.
3. Add lavender essential oil if desired for its calming and soothing skin benefits.
4. Pour the mixture into a small tin or jar and let it solidify at room temperature.
5. To use, apply a small amount of the balm to areas of the skin that are exposed to environmental stressors, such as the face, hands, and neck.
6. Use daily, especially before going outside, to protect the skin from pollution, UV rays, and other harmful environmental factors.

Nutritional Values (per serving):

- Ricinoleic Acid: Offers anti-inflammatory and hydrating properties.
- Fatty Acids in Shea Butter: Help fortify the skin's moisture barrier.

Castor and Rosewater Hydrating Mist- Refreshes and Hydrates All Day

Ingredients:

- 2 tablespoons castor oil.
- 1 /4 cup rosewater.
- Optional: 2 drops of glycerin for added moisture retention.

Instructions:

1. In a clean spray bottle, combine the castor oil and rosewater Castor oil helps to hydrate and lock in moisture, while rosewater tones and refreshes the skin.
2. Add glycerin if using; it acts as a humectant to further help the skin retain moisture.
3. Shake the bottle vigorously to ensure all ingredients are well mixed.
4. To use, spritz the hydrating mist lightly over your face whenever your skin feels dry or needs refreshing It can be applied over makeup or on bare skin.
5. Use throughout the day for a quick, refreshing, and hydrating boost.

Nutritional Values (per serving):

- Ricinoleic Acid: Provides hydration and helps maintain skin moisture.
- Rosewater: Offers natural anti-inflammatory properties and soothes the skin.

Detoxifying Castor and Coffee Scrub - Invigorates and Smooths Skin

Ingredients:

- 2 tablespoons castor oil.
- 1 / 4 cup ground coffee.
- 1 tablespoon coconut oil.

Instructions:

1. In a mixing bowl, combine the ground coffee, castor oil, and coconut oil Coffee is excellent for exfoliation and boosting circulation, while castor and coconut oils provide moisture.
2. Mix all ingredients together until you have a coarse paste.
3. To use, apply the scrub to damp skin in the shower, massaging in circular

motions to exfoliate and invigorate the skin.

4. Rinse off thoroughly with warm water The scrub not only smooths and refines skin texture but also helps to flush out toxins and improve circulation.
5. Use once or twice a week for best results.

Nutritional Values (per serving):

- Ricinoleic Acid: Moisturizes and promotes a healthy skin barrier.
- Caffeine: Known for its anti-inflammatory and firming properties.

Soothing Castor and Chamomile Night Lotion - For Sensitive and Irritated Skin

Ingredients:

- 2 tablespoons castor oil.
- 1 /4 cup chamomile tea (cooled).
- 1 tablespoon shea butter.

Instructions:

1. Brew a strong chamomile tea and allow it to cool completely.
2. In a double boiler, melt the shea butter.
3. Once melted, remove from heat and mix in the castor oil and the cooled chamomile tea.
4. Stir until all ingredients are fully incorporated and begin to thicken as they cool.
5. Transfer the lotion to a clean container with a lid.
6. To use, apply the lotion to clean skin at night, focusing on areas that are particularly sensitive or irritated.
7. The soothing properties of chamomile and the hydrating effects of castor oil work overnight to calm and restore skin.

Nutritional Values (per serving):

- Ricinoleic Acid: Calms inflammation and hydrates the skin.

- Chamomile: Contains anti-inflammatory and antioxidant properties ideal for soothing sensitive skin.

CHAPTER 4

CASTOR OIL FOR HAIR HEALTH

The Basics of Natural Hair Care

Using materials straight from nature, natural hair care is all about appreciating the health and originality of your hair. These practices prioritize gentle treatments and avoid harsh chemicals, ensuring that the hair remains strong, nourished, and vibrant. One of the key components in the arsenal of natural hair care is castor oil, a versatile oil known for its remarkable benefits for scalp health and hair growth.

At the heart of natural hair care lies the principle of minimalism and safety, focusing on what is truly beneficial for hair health. The focus is on staying away from artificial substances that deplete hair of its natural oils, causing breakage and dryness. Instead, natural hair care promotes the use of products that mimic the hair's natural sebum, with castor oil being a prime example due to its rich, moisturizing properties.

Rich in fatty acids, especially ricinoleic acid, castor oil is made from the seeds of the castor bean plant. It is thick and sticky. This unique composition makes it highly prized in natural hair care routines. It is well known that ricinoleic acid lubricates the hair shaft, promoting elasticity and lowering breakage risk. Additionally, castor oil is rich in nutrients, fortifies the hair's roots, and nourishes the scalp.

One of the foremost benefits of castor oil is its ability to promote a healthier scalp. The basis for good hair development is a healthy scalp.

Castor oil's anti-inflammatory properties help soothe irritated and itchy scalps, reducing dandruff and other scalp disorders. This creates a healthier environment for hair follicles, which is essential for optimal hair growth. The oil's antimicrobial properties also help protect the scalp from bacterial and fungal infections, which can affect scalp health and impede hair growth.

Furthermore, castor oil is renowned for its ability to stimulate hair growth. The mechanism behind this is thought to be linked to its ability to improve circulation to the scalp. Improved blood flow ensures that hair follicles receive more of the nutrients necessary to stimulate growth. Regular application of castor oil has been reported to enhance the thickness and density of hair, as the oil not only promotes growth but also helps in reducing hair loss by strengthening the roots.

Incorporating castor oil into a natural hair care routine can be done in several ways. One common method is the scalp massage. Massaging the scalp with castor oil helps invigorate the scalp, improving circulation and promoting healthier hair growth. This method also ensures that the oil deeply penetrates the scalp, moisturizing it and boosting the overall health of the hair follicles.

Another popular use of castor oil is in homemade hair masks. A typical hair mask might include castor oil mixed with another lighter oil, such as coconut or olive oil, to enhance manageability and spread ability. Ingredients like honey or aloe vera might be added for their additional hydrating and healing properties. These masks are usually applied to the hair and left on for a period before washing out, leaving the hair intensely nourished and rejuvenated.

The benefits of using castor oil in natural hair care are extensive, ranging from improved hair texture and increased growth to a healthier scalp. Those who switch to this natural approach often notice a significant improvement not only in the health of their hair but also in its appearance.

Hair becomes more resilient, shinier, and thicker, with the soothing effects of the oil bringing added comfort to the scalp.

Adopting castor oil as a key element in your hair care regimen can transform your hair's health. By aligning with the principles of natural hair care, castor oil helps foster a holistic approach to beauty, focusing on long-term health and the preservation of your hair's natural vitality. As we continue to understand more about the benefits of natural ingredients, castor oil stands out as a testament to the power of nature in enhancing our beauty naturally and effectively.

Scientific Studies about castor oil for Hair Care

While castor oil has long been celebrated in traditional remedies for its extensive benefits to hair health, its effectiveness is further bolstered by scientific research. Numerous studies have delved into how castor oil contributes to hair growth and scalp health, unveiling the biological mechanisms behind its benefits. This scientific exploration into castor oil's role in hair care provides not just anecdotal but solid, scientifically supported reasons for its use in maintaining healthy hair and scalp.

About 90% of castor oil is made up of the fatty acid ricinoleic acid, which is one of the main ingredients that has drawn the interest of scientists. The anti-inflammatory qualities of ricinoleic acid are well-known, and they are essential for preserving scalp health. Dandruff and other scalp problems that damage hair follicles or interfere with the hair's natural development cycle can be caused by inflammation of the scalp, which can also prevent hair growth. By mitigating inflammation, castor oil helps maintain a healthy scalp environment conducive to hair growth.

Research has indicated that the anti-inflammatory characteristics of castor oil are a result of its capacity to lower the body's levels of prostaglandin

E2 (PGE2). PGE2 is associated with inflammatory processes in the body, and its reduction can, therefore, help control such responses on the scalp. A study published in the "Journal of Lipid Research" highlighted how ricinoleic acid inhibits the production of PGE2, providing a biochemical basis for the traditional use of castor oil in treating scalp inflammation.

Additionally, castor oil is believed to enhance blood circulation to the scalp, which is another crucial factor in promoting hair growth. More nutrients and oxygen are provided to the hair follicles through improved blood flow, which is necessary for healthy hair development. While direct studies on castor oil increasing blood circulation in the scalp are limited, the general pharmacological effects of ricinoleic acid include vessel dilation, which can improve blood flow. This theory is supported by the empirical benefits reported in multiple user testimonials and aligns with known properties of other similar fatty acids.

Castor oil's role in moisturizing the hair and scalp also contributes significantly to its effectiveness in hair care. Given that it is a humectant, moisture is retained by halting the loss of water through the skin's outer layer. This property not only improves hair elasticity, reducing the risk of breakage but also maintains a hydrated scalp, thereby reducing flakiness and dry scalp conditions. A study published in the "International Journal of Trichology" explored various natural oils and highlighted how oils like castor oil, which are rich in fatty acids, provide essential nutrients to hair follicles and prevent scalp dryness.

The ability of castor oil to combat fungal infections, such as those caused by the dandruff fcausing fungus Malassezia, further underscores its utility in hair care. The antimicrobial properties of castor oil, although more broadly studied in skin applications, suggest similar benefits when applied to the scalp. This aligns with anecdotal evidence and traditional uses, implying that regular application of castor oil could contribute to a healthier scalp, free from microbial infections that could otherwise compromise hair health.

15 Nourishing Castor Oil Recipes for Hair Growth and Scalp Health

Basic Castor Oil Scalp Massage - Stimulates hair follicles for growth

Ingredients:

- 2 tablespoons castor oil.
- 1 tablespoon coconut oil (optional for added moisture and easier application).
- Optional: 5 drops of peppermint essential oil (for enhanced stimulation and freshness).

Instructions:

1. In a small bowl, mix the castor oil with coconut oil if using Coconut oil helps to lighten the texture of castor oil, making it easier to apply and rinse out It also adds additional moisturizing benefits.
2. Add the peppermint essential oil if desired Peppermint oil is known for its invigorating and stimulating properties, which can enhance the massage and promote blood circulation to the scalp.
3. Stir the oils together until well combined.

Nutritional Values (per serving):

- Ricinoleic Acid: 90% of castor oil, known for anti-inflammatory and antimicrobial properties
- Lauric Acid: Found in coconut oil, provides deep conditioning and helps prevent protein loss.

- Menthol: Present in peppermint oil, enhances blood flow and provides a cooling sensation.

Castor and Coconut Oil Hair Mask - Deeply Moisturizes and Strengthens Hair

Ingredients:

- 2 tablespoons castor oil
- 2 tablespoons coconut oil
- 1 tablespoon honey (optional for added hydration and shine)

Instructions:

1. In a small mixing bowl, combine the castor oil and coconut oil Coconut oil is solid at room temperature, so you may need to gently warm it to a liquid state before mixing.
2. If desired, add honey to the mixture Honey is a natural humectant that helps attract moisture to the hair and adds a healthy shine.
3. Stir all the ingredients together until they are well blended and smooth.

Nutritional Values (per serving):

- Ricinoleic Acid: Moisturizes and reduces scalp inflammation.
- Lauric Acid: Found in coconut oil, helps strengthen the hair and reduce protein loss.
- Enzymes and Nutrients in Honey: Adds hydration and shine.

Rosemary and Castor Oil Blend - Enhances

Circulation and Promotes Growth

Ingredients:

- 2 tablespoons castor oil.
- 1 tablespoon rosemary essential oil.
- 1 tablespoon olive oil (optional for added nourishment).

Instructions:

1. In a small bowl, combine the castor oil and rosemary essential oil Rosemary oil is known for its ability to stimulate blood circulation, which can promote hair growth.
2. If desired, add olive oil to the mixture Olive oil is rich in antioxidants and provides additional nourishment and shine to the hair.
3. Mix the oils thoroughly to ensure they are well combined.

Nutritional Values (per serving):

- Ricinoleic Acid: Anti-inflammatory and promotes healthy hair growth.
- Antioxidants in Rosemary Oil: Stimulate blood circulation and promote hair growth.
- Oleic Acid in Olive Oil: Adds moisture and shine to the hair.

Peppermint and Castor Oil Scalp Treatment - Invigorates Scalp for Healthy Hair

Ingredients:

- 2 tablespoons castor oil.
- 1tablespoon coconut oil (optional for easier application).
- 5 drops peppermint essential oil.

Instructions:

1. In a small mixing bowl, combine castor oil and coconut oil if using Coconut oil helps to lighten the texture of castor oil, making it easier to apply.
2. Add peppermint essential oil to the mixture Peppermint oil is known for its invigorating properties and ability to stimulate blood circulation.
3. Stir the oils together until well combined.

Nutritional Values (per serving):

- Ricinoleic Acid: Known for its anti-inflammatory and antimicrobial properties.
- Lauric Acid: Found in coconut oil, provides deep conditioning and helps prevent protein loss.
- Menthol: Present in peppermint oil, enhances blood flow and provides a cooling sensation.

Tea Tree and Castor Oil Anti-Dandruff Serum - Soothes and Clears Flaky Scalp

Ingredients:

- 2 tablespoons castor oil.
- 1 tablespoon jojoba oil.
- 5 drops tea tree essential oil.

Instructions:

1. In a small mixing bowl, combine castor oil and jojoba oil Jojoba oil is a lightweight oil that helps to balance the scalp's natural oils.
2. Add tea tree essential oil to the mixture Tea tree oil is known for its antifungal and antibacterial properties, making it effective against dandruff
3. Stir the oils together until well combined

- Ricinoleic Acid: Anti-inflammatory and promotes healthy hair growth.
- Oleic Acid in Jojoba Oil: Helps balance the scalp's natural oils.
- Terpinenol: Active ingredient in tea tree oil, known for combating pathogens that cause dandruff.

Castor and Jojoba Oil Hair Serum - Balances Oil Production and Nourishes Roots

Ingredients:

- 2 tablespoons castor oil
- 2 tablespoons jojoba oil
- Optional: 5 drops rosemary essential oil for added hair growth benefits

Instructions:

1. In a small mixing bowl, combine castor oil and jojoba oil Jojoba oil closely mimics the scalp's natural sebum, making it effective in balancing oil production.
2. If desired, add rosemary essential oil to enhance hair growth.
3. Stir the oils together until well combined.
4. Transfer the serum into a clean glass bottle with a dropper for easy application.

Nutritional Values (per serving):

- Ricinoleic Acid: Anti-inflammatory and antimicrobial properties.
- Oleic Acid in Jojoba Oil: Balances scalp's natural oils and provides moisture.

Lavender and Castor Oil Night Treatment- Calms

Scalp and Encourages Thickness

Ingredients:

- 2 tablespoons castor oil.
- 2 tablespoons almond oil.
- 5 drops lavender essential oil.

Instructions:

1. In a small mixing bowl, combine castor oil and almond oil Almond oil is light and penetrates the hair shaft easily, providing deep nourishment.
2. Add lavender essential oil to the mixture for its calming and hair thickening properties
3. Stir the oils together until well combined.
4. Transfer the treatment into a clean glass bottle with a dropper for easy application.

Nutritional Values (per serving):

- Ricinoleic Acid: Anti-inflammatory and promotes hair growth.
- Vitamin E in Almond Oil: Provides antioxidant protection and moisturizes the scalp.

Castor Oil and Egg Protein Mask- Repairs and Strengthens Hair Strands

Ingredients:

- 2 tablespoons castor oil.
- 1 egg (rich in protein).
- 1 tablespoon olive oil (optional for added moisture).

Instructions:

1. In a small mixing bowl, whisk the egg until it is well beaten.
2. Add castor oil and olive oil to the egg, mixing

thoroughly to create a smooth consistency.

3. Stir the ingredients until well combined.

Nutritional Values (per serving):

- Ricinoleic Acid: Anti-inflammatory and promotes hair growth.
- Proteins in Egg: Strengthen hair strands and repair damage.
- Oleic Acid in Olive Oil: Adds moisture and shine to hair.

Castor and Aloe Vera Scalp Gel - Hydrates and Soothes the Scalp

Ingredients:

- 2 tablespoons castor oil.
- 2 tablespoons aloe vera gel.
- 5 drops tea tree essential oil (optional for added soothing properties).

Instructions:

1. In a small mixing bowl, combine castor oil and aloe vera gel Aloe vera gel is known for its hydrating and soothing properties.
2. If desired, add tea tree essential oil for its antifungal and soothing effects.
3. Stir the ingredients together until well blended and smooth.

Nutritional Values (per serving):

- Ricinoleic Acid: Known for its anti-inflammatory and antimicrobial properties.
- Vitamins and Enzymes in Aloe Vera: Hydrate and soothe the scalp.

Yogurt and Castor Oil Hair Conditioner - Smooths and Detangles Hair

Ingredients:

- 2 tablespoons castor oil.
- 1 /2 cup plain yogurt.
- 1 tablespoon honey (optional for added moisture and shine).

Instructions:

1. In a small mixing bowl, combine castor oil and plain yogurt is rich in proteins and lactic acid, which help to condition and detangle hair.
2. If desired, add honey to the mixture for its moisturizing and shine enhancing properties.
3. Stir all the ingredients together until well combined and smooth.

Nutritional Values (per serving):

- Ricinoleic Acid: Anti-inflammatory and promotes hair growth.
- Proteins and Lactic Acid in Yogurt: Condition and detangle hair.
- Enzymes and Nutrients in Honey: Adds hydration and shine.

Hibiscus and Castor Oil Hair Tonic - Boosts Shine and Over-all Hair Health

Ingredients:

- 2 tablespoons castor oil.
- 1 / 2 cup hibiscus tea (cooled).
- 1 tablespoon apple cider vinegar (optional for added shine).

Instructions:

1. Brew a strong hibiscus tea and allow it to cool completely.
2. In a small mixing bowl, combine castor oil and the cooled hibiscus tea Hibiscus is rich in

antioxidants and vitamins that promote hair health.
3. If desired, add apple cider vinegar to the mixture for its shine enhancing properties.
4. Stir the ingredients together until well combined.

Nutritional Values (per serving):

- Ricinoleic Acid: Anti-inflammatory and promotes hair growth
- Antioxidants in Hibiscus: Boosts hair health and shine.
- Acetic Acid in Apple Cider Vinegar: Adds shine and balances scalp pH.

Castor and Argan Oil Leave - In Conditioner Protects and Softens Hair

Ingredients:

- 2 tablespoons castor oil.
- 2 tablespoons argan oil.
- Optional: 5 drops lavender essential oil for added scent and calming properties.

Instructions:

1. In a small mixing bowl, combine castor oil and argan oil Argan oil is known for its light texture and high vitamin E content, which helps to protect and nourish hair.
2. If desired, add lavender essential oil to the mixture for a pleasant scent and additional calming benefits.
3. Stir the oils together until well combined.
4. Transfer the mixture to a clean glass bottle with a spray nozzle or a pump for easy application.

Nutritional Values (per serving):

- Ricinoleic Acid: Provides deep hydration and anti-inflammatory benefits.

- Vitamin E in Argan Oil: Protects hair from environmental damage and adds shine.

Ginger and Castor Oil Scalp Activator -Stimulates Hair Follicles for New Growth

Ingredients:

- 2 tablespoons castor oil.
- 1 tablespoon ginger juice (freshly grated and squeezed ginger).
- Optional: 5 drops peppermint essential oil for enhanced stimulation.

Instructions:

1. In a small mixing bowl, combine castor oil and fresh ginger juice Ginger juice is known for its stimulating properties that can promote hair growth.
2. If desired, add peppermint essential oil to the mixture for a cooling sensation and added stimulation.
3. Stir the ingredients together until well combined.

Nutritional Values (per serving):

- Ricinoleic Acid: Anti-inflammatory and promotes hair growth.
- Gingerol in Ginger Juice: Stimulates blood circulation and promotes hair growth.

Castor and Apple Cider Vinegar Scalp Cleanser- Clarifies and Restores Scalp Health

Ingredients:

- 2 tablespoons castor oil.

- 1 /4 cup apple cider vinegar.
- 1 /2 cup distilled water.

Instructions:

1. In a small mixing bowl, combine castor oil, apple cider vinegar, and distilled water Apple cider vinegar is known for its clarifying properties and ability to balance scalp pH.
2. Stir the ingredients together until well combined
3. Transfer the mixture to a clean bottle with a nozzle for easy application.

Nutritional Values (per serving):

- Ricinoleic Acid: Provides deep hydration and anti-inflammatory benefits.
- Acetic Acid in Apple Cider Vinegar: Clarifies and balances scalp Ph.

Castor and Olive Oil Hot Oil Treatment -

Penetrates Deeply for Ultimate Nourishment

Ingredients:

- 2 tablespoons castor oil.
- 2 tablespoons olive oil.
- Optional: 5 drops rosemary essential oil for added hair growth benefits.

Instructions:

1. In a small heat safe bowl, combine castor oil and olive oil Olive oil is rich in antioxidants and deeply penetrates the hair shaft for ultimate nourishment.
2. If desired, add rosemary essential oil to the mixture for additional hair growth benefits.
3. Warm the mixture gently in a microwave or using a double boiler until it is comfortably warm to the touch.

Nutritional Values (per serving):

- Ricinoleic Acid: Anti-inflammatory and promotes hair growth.

- Oleic Acid in Olive Oil: Deeply moisturizes and nourishes hair.

We're Halfway There!

Thank you for continuing to read our book We hope you're finding it useful and enjoyable Your feedback is essential for us to keep providing high-quality content

Why Your Review Matters:

By leaving a review, you help us understand how we can improve and what you enjoyed the most Your feedback is also crucial for other readers who are considering this book

How You Can Share Your Review:

Through Amazon.com:
- Go to the Amazon page where you found my book
- Navigate to the 'Customer Reviews' section
- Click on 'Write a customer review' to share your valuable insights

Instant QR Code Access: Simply scan the QR code below with your smartphone to be directed to the Amazon review section

Thank you for your continued support!

CHAPTER 5
REMEDIES FOR JOINT AND MUSCLE

Castor Oil for Pain Relief: Joint and Muscle Treatments

Castor oil is a well-liked option for natural pain relief, especially in the treatment of joint and muscular pain, because of its well established potent anti-inflammatory qualities. Castor oil is derived from the seeds of the Ricinus communis plant and includes ricinoleic acid, a fatty acid with anti-inflammatory properties. This is the main ingredient in castor oil, which has topical pain and inflammation relieving properties.

The process of using castor oil for pain relief involves its application as a topical massage oil or through the use of castor oil packs. When massaged directly onto the skin over affected areas, castor oil penetrates deeply into the tissues. The ricinoleic acid in the oil then works to inhibit the production of certain chemicals in the body involved in the inflammatory process, such as prostaglandins. This activity aids in the reduction of pain, stiffness, and inflammation brought on by ailments, including rheumatism, arthritis, and muscular soreness.

In addition to direct application, castor oil packs are another common method for treating joint and muscle pain. To prepare a castor oil pack, the oil is soaked into a piece of cloth, which is then placed directly on the skin over the painful area. Use a hot water bottle or heating pad to impart heat to the fabric and cover it with plastic wrap to increase the therapy's effectiveness. The heat promotes blood flow to the region, which facilitates ricinoleic acid's deeper tissue penetration and amplifies the anti-inflammatory properties of the oil.

The benefits of using castor oil for pain relief also extend to its moisturizing properties, which help maintain smooth and supple skin, further facilitating the massage process. Moreover, the soothing nature of the oil makes the massage experience itself quite therapeutic, contributing to overall relaxation and a reduction in pain perception.

Research supporting the use of castor oil for pain relief primarily points to its anti-inflammatory capabilities. According to studies, castor oil can effectively alleviate pain and inflammation when used topically without having the negative side effects that are sometimes connected to prescription painkillers. This makes it a worthwhile choice for anybody looking for a pain reduction strategy that is all natural.

Overall, castor oil is a beneficial and versatile oil for the management of joint and muscle pain. Its natural anti-inflammatory properties, combined with the ease of application either directly or through oil packs, make it a practical and effective natural remedy for reducing pain and enhancing joint and muscle function. Whether used alone or in conjunction with other treatments, castor oil can provide significant relief for those suffering from chronic pain or temporary discomfort due to muscle tension or injuries.

Scientific Studies about castor oil for Joint and Muscle Treatments

Castor oil has been traditionally used for its therapeutic benefits in relieving joint and muscle pain, but it is the scientific backing that really highlights its efficacy. Several studies have examined how castor oil can be beneficial in these applications, focusing particularly on its anti-inflammatory and analgesic properties.

Ricinoleic acid, the primary constituent of castor oil, has been found to possess strong anti-inflammatory properties. A study published in the **Journal of Ethnopharmacology** examined the anti-inflammatory effects of ricinoleic acid and found that it significantly reduces inflammation when applied topically. This action is largely due to its ability to inhibit the release of proinflammatory substances in the body, such as prostaglandins, which are often associated with pain and inflammation in joints and muscles.

Further research in the **International Journal of Pharmaceutical Sciences and Research** explored the transdermal absorption of ricinoleic acid, noting its effective penetration through the skin barrier. This property is crucial for the treatment of deep tissue pain, such as that found in muscles and joints, as it allows the active components of castor oil to reach the affected areas more effectively.

Its impact on lymphatic circulation has also supported castor oil's benefits for joint and muscle treatments. A study highlighted in the **Alternative Medicine Review** noted that castor oil packs—fabric soaked in castor oil placed on the skin with applied heat—promote lymphatic circulation. This can reduce the buildup of toxins and inflammatory components in joint and muscle tissues, thereby alleviating pain and swelling.

Moreover, the analgesic (pain-relieving) properties of castor oil have been observed in various anecdotal evidence and smaller-scale studies. While largescale clinical trials are still needed to define the scope of castor oil's effectiveness conclusively, the existing research provides a strong foundation for its use in treating joint and muscle discomfort.

In practical applications, patients with arthritis and other chronic inflammatory conditions have reported significant relief from pain and improved mobility after using castor oil either in massages or as part of castor oil packs. The warming sensation provided by the packs, combined with the oil's natural properties, helps to soothe stiff muscles and painful joints, further enhancing its therapeutic benefits.

5 Castor Oil Remedies for Pain Management

Warming Castor Oil & Cayenne Salve

Ingredients:

- 2 tablespoons castor oil.
- 2 tablespoons coconut oil.
- 1 tablespoon beeswax.
- 1 teaspoon cayenne pepper powder.
- Optional: 5 drops of ginger essential oil for added warmth.

Instructions:

- In a double boiler, melt the beeswax and coconut oil together until fully liquid.
- Remove from heat and stir in the castor oil and cayenne pepper powder.
- If desired, add ginger essential oil for additional warming effects.

- Pour the mixture into a small glass jar and let it cool until it solidifies.
- To use, apply a small amount of the salve to the affected area and gently massage it in.

Nutritional Values (per serving):

- Ricinoleic Acid: Known for its anti-inflammatory and analgesic properties.
- Capsaicin in Cayenne Pepper: Provides a warming effect that helps to relieve pain.
- Lauric Acid in Coconut Oil: Adds moisturizing and antimicrobial benefits

Turmeric and Castor Oil Compress

Ingredients:

- 2 tablespoons castor oil.
- 1 teaspoon turmeric powder.
- 1 tablespoon aloe vera gel.
- A piece of flannel or cotton cloth.

Instructions:

- In a small bowl, mix castor oil, turmeric powder, and aloe vera gel until well combined.
- Apply the mixture to the affected area.
- Cover the area with the flannel or cotton cloth.
- Place a heating pad or hot water bottle over the cloth to provide gentle heat.
- Leave the compress on for 20-30 minutes.

Nutritional Values (per serving):

- Ricinoleic Acid: Anti-inflammatory and analgesic properties.
- Curcumin in Turmeric: Provides powerful anti-inflammatory benefits.
- Enzymes and Vitamins in Aloe Vera: Hydrate and soothe the skin.

Lavender Infused Castor Oil Massage Blend

Ingredients:

- 2 tablespoons castor oil.
- 1 tablespoon sweet almond oil.
- 10 drops lavender essential oil.

Instructions:

- In a small bottle, combine castor oil and sweet almond oil.
- Add lavender essential oil and shake well to mix.
- Warm the oil blend slightly before use for enhanced relaxation.
- Massage the oil blend into the affected area using gentle, circular motions.

Nutritional Values (per serving):

- Ricinoleic Acid: Anti-inflammatory and promotes healing.
- Oleic Acid in Sweet Almond Oil: Provides deep moisture and nourishment.
- Linalool in Lavender Oil: Offers calming and anti-inflammatory properties.

Eucalyptus & Castor Oil Muscle Rub

Ingredients:

- 2 tablespoons castor oil.
- 2 tablespoons olive oil.
- 10 drops eucalyptus essential oil.

Instructions:

- In a small bowl, mix castor oil and olive oil.
- Add eucalyptus essential oil and stir well.
- Warm the mixture slightly before applying.

- Apply the rub to the sore muscles and massage it in gently.

Nutritional Values (per serving):

- Ricinoleic Acid: Provides anti-inflammatory and analgesic benefits.
- Oleic Acid in Olive Oil: Deeply moisturizes and nourishes the skin.
- Eucalyptol in Eucalyptus Oil: Provides anti-inflammatory and analgesic effects.

Peppermint Castor Oil Joint Therapy

Ingredients:

- 2 tablespoons castor oil.
- 1 tablespoon jojoba oil.
- 10 drops peppermint essential oil.

Instructions:

- In a small bottle, combine castor oil and jojoba oil.
- Add peppermint essential oil and shake well to mix.
- Apply the mixture to the joints and massage gently.
- Use a heating pad after application for enhanced relief.

Nutritional Values (per serving):

- Ricinoleic Acid: Anti-inflammatory and analgesic properties.
- Oleic Acid in Jojoba Oil: Balances and hydrates the skin.
- Menthol in Peppermint Oil: Provides a cooling and numbing effect.

CHAPTER 6
REMEDIES FOR DIGESTIVE HEALTH

Digestive Health: How to Safely Use Castor Oil Internally

Castor oil, known for its powerful laxative properties, has been a traditional remedy for various digestive issues, including constipation. It works by stimulating the muscles that push material through the intestines, effectively clearing the bowels. This action is primarily due to the ricinoleic acid in castor oil, which binds to muscle cells in the intestinal walls, causing contractions that facilitate stool movement.

Despite its effectiveness, castor oil must be used with great caution when taken internally for digestive health. Castor oil can interact with other drugs, so it's important to first speak with a healthcare practitioner, especially if you have any preexisting medical issues or are taking any other prescriptions.

When taking a single dose, people should usually consume between 15 and 60 milliliters. It is crucial not to exceed this dosage or use castor oil frequently, as overuse can lead to significant health issues, including electrolyte imbalances and chronic constipation. Frequent use may also cause dependence on laxatives for bowel movements.

Given that castor oil can stimulate contractions in the muscles, which may have an impact on the uterus, it is not advised for pregnant women to use it. Castor oil can cause newborns to throw up in their breast milk; therefore, nursing moms should also stay away from it. When considering castor oil for children, a pediatrician's consultation is essential to adjust the dosage appropriately.

Possible side effects of taking castor oil internally include abdominal cramping, nausea, diarrhea, and dizziness. Dehydration and electrolyte imbalances brought on by severe diarrhea can be dangerous for the elderly and people with weakened immune systems.

It is best to consume castor oil on an empty stomach to maximize its efficiency and absorption. The effects typically occur within two to six hours, so it is advisable to remain at home and close to a bathroom after ingestion.

Castor oil should not be used continuously for more than seven days, as prolonged use can reduce natural bowel function and lead to a loss of muscle tone in the bowels.

Scientific Studies about castor oil for internal use

Castor oil, primarily valued for its effective laxative properties, has been the subject of various scientific studies that explore its internal use. The key active component, ricinoleic acid, is released in the intestine and stimulates the smooth muscle cells of the intestinal walls. This action induces strong laxative effects by increasing intestinal movements, thereby facilitating bowel movements. The research highlighted in the Journal of Ethnopharmacology points to ricinoleic acid's role in activating receptors on muscle cells in the intestines, leading to these powerful contractions.

Castor oil is being studied for its anti-inflammatory properties beyond its laxative application; these properties may be especially helpful for illnesses like inflammatory bowel disease (IBD). According to studies published in Digestive Diseases and Sciences, castor oil can reduce inflammation in the gut mucosa, which is crucial for alleviating symptoms of IBD. This suggests that castor oil could complement traditional therapies for IBD, offering a natural treatment option with anti-inflammatory benefits.

However, the safety and potential toxicity of castor oil cannot be overlooked. The International Journal of Toxicology provides a comprehensive review of castor oil's safety profile, noting that while it is generally safe in limited dosages, excessive use can lead to serious side effects such as electrolyte imbalances, dehydration, and even an increased risk of cardiac arrhythmias due to significant losses of potassium and other electrolytes.

Further research in the American Journal of Clinical Nutrition explores how castor oil affects the absorption of nutrients in the gut. The findings indicate that although castor oil increases the transit time through the intestine, it does not significantly impair the absorption of nutrients, suggesting that its use for constipation does not adversely affect nutritional status.

Medical guidelines advocate for castor oil to be used only as a shortterm treatment for constipation, recommending a single dose of up to 1560 milliliters for adults, which is considered safe for occasional use. These guidelines also caution against habitual use due to the risks of dependency and the side effects mentioned above.

Overall, while the benefits of castor oil for internal use, especially as a laxative and for its anti-inflammatory properties, are supported by scientific evidence, the need for careful and informed usage is clear. Castor oil's therapeutic potential and safety profile need to be further clarified via ongoing research and clinical studies before it can be utilized in medicine with confidence.

10 Castor Oil Internal Use Formulas for Digestive Health

Soothing Castor & Ginger Laxative Tea

Ingredients:
- 1 tablespoon castor oil.
- 1 teaspoon freshly grated ginger.
- 1 cup hot water.
- 1 teaspoon honey (optional)

Instructions:
1. Grate fresh ginger and place it in a cup.
2. Pour hot water over the ginger and let it steep for 5 minutes.
3. Strain the ginger tea into another cup.
4. Add castor oil to the ginger tea and stir well.
5. If desired, add honey to sweeten.
6. Drink the tea in the morning on an empty stomach for best results.

Nutritional Values (per serving):
- Ricinoleic Acid: Anti-inflammatory and laxative properties.
- Gingerol in Ginger: Aids digestion and reduces nausea.
- Honey: Provides soothing and antimicrobial benefits.

Lemon Castor Oil Morning Detox

Ingredients:
- 1 tablespoon castor oil.
- Juice of 1 lemon.
- 1 cup warm water.

Instructions:
1. Squeeze the juice of one lemon into a cup of warm water.
2. Add castor oil and stir well.
3. Drink the mixture in the morning on an empty stomach.

Nutritional Values (per serving):
- Ricinoleic Acid: Promotes bowel movements.
- Vitamin C in Lemon Juice: Boosts immune system and aids detoxification.

Orange Juice & Castor Oil Constipation Relief

Ingredients:
- 1 tablespoon castor oil.
- 1 cup fresh orange juice.

Instructions:
1. Pour fresh orange juice into a glass.
2. Add castor oil and stir well.
3. Drink the mixture in the morning on an empty stomach.

Nutritional Values (per serving):
1. Ricinoleic Acid: Stimulates bowel movements.
2. Vitamin C and Fiber in Orange Juice: Support digestive health.

Digestive Wellness Castor Oil Smoothie

Ingredients:

- 1 tablespoon castor oil.
- 1 cup almond milk.
- 1 banana.
- 1 tablespoon chia seeds.
- 1 teaspoon honey (optional)

Instructions:

1. In a blender, combine almond milk, banana, chia seeds, and honey.
2. Add castor oil and blend until smooth.
3. Drink the smoothie in the morning for a nutritious start to your day.

Nutritional Values (per serving):

- Ricinoleic Acid: Helps relieve constipation
- Fiber in Banana and Chia Seeds: Supports digestive health
- Almond Milk: Provides hydration and nutrients

Mint-Infused Castor Oil Capsules

Ingredients:

- 1 tablespoon castor oil.
- 23 drops peppermint essential oil.
- Gel capsules.

Instructions:

1. Mix castor oil with peppermint essential oil.
2. Using a dropper, fill the gel capsules with the mixture.
3. Take 12 capsules with a glass of water.

Nutritional Values (per serving):

Ricinoleic Acid: Laxative properties

Menthol in Peppermint Oil: Soothes the digestive tract

Pineapple & Castor Oil Anti-Bloat Drink

Ingredients:
- 1 tablespoon castor oil
- 1 cup fresh pineapple juice

Instructions:
1. Pour fresh pineapple juice into a glass.
2. Add castor oil and stir well.
3. Drink the mixture to help reduce bloating.

Nutritional Values (per serving):
- Ricinoleic Acid: Relieves constipation
- Bromelain in Pineapple Juice: Aids digestion and reduces bloating

Turmeric & Castor Oil Digestive Aid

Ingredients:
- 1 tablespoon castor oil
- 1 teaspoon turmeric powder
- 1 cup warm water

Instructions:
1. Mix turmeric powder into a cup of warm water.
2. Add castor oil and stir well.
3. Drink the mixture for digestive relief.

Nutritional Values (per serving):
- Ricinoleic Acid: Anti-inflammatory and laxative properties
- Curcumin in Turmeric: Provides anti-inflammatory benefits

Herbal Tea with Castor Oil for Gut Health

Ingredients:
- 1 tablespoon castor oil
- 1 cup brewed herbal tea (chamomile, peppermint, or ginger)

Instructions:

1. Brew your favorite herbal tea and let it cool slightly.
2. Add castor oil and stir well.
3. Drink the tea for digestive health benefits.

Nutritional Values (per serving):

- Ricinoleic Acid: Promotes bowel movements
- Herbal Tea Compounds: Soothe the digestive tract

Prune & Castor Oil Digestive Elixir

Ingredients:

- 1 tablespoon castor oil
- 1 cup prune juice

Instructions:

1. Pour prune juice into a glass.
2. Add castor oil and stir well.
3. Drink the mixture for a potent digestive aid.

Nutritional Values (per serving):

- Ricinoleic Acid: Stimulates bowel movements
- Fiber in Prune Juice: Supports regular bowel movements

Warm Milk & Castor Oil Laxative Mix

Ingredients:

- 1 tablespoon castor oil
- 1 cup warm milk
- 1 teaspoon honey (optional)

Instructions:

1. Warm the milk and pour it into a cup.
2. Add castor oil and stir well.
3. If desired, add honey for taste.
4. Drink the mixture before bedtime for overnight relief.

Nutritional Values (per serving):

- Ricinoleic Acid: Laxative properties
- Calcium in Milk: Supports bone health
- Honey: Provides soothing benefits

CHAPTER 7
ETHICAL AND SUSTAINABLE PRACTICES

Choosing Ethically Sourced Castor Oil

Choosing ethically sourced castor oil is crucial for ensuring that the benefits of this versatile product extend beyond personal health and wellness. Ethically sourced castor oil not only provides quality assurance but also supports sustainable farming practices, protects the environment, and improves the livelihoods of local communities involved in its production. This discussion delves into the importance of ethically sourcing castor oil and its broader impact on both local communities and the environment.

Ethically sourced castor oil ensures that the farming practices used in its cultivation are sustainable and environmentally friendly. Chemical pesticides and fertilizers are frequently used in conventional farming practices, which can degrade soil, contaminate water supplies, and reduce biodiversity. In contrast, sustainable farming practices prioritize the use of organic fertilizers, crop rotation, and other ecofriendly techniques that maintain soil health and preserve local ecosystems. By choosing castor oil from suppliers who use sustainable methods, consumers can help reduce the environmental footprint of castor oil production and promote agricultural practices that are better for the planet.

The production of castor oil has significant implications for local communities, especially in regions where castor beans are a primary crop. In many developing countries, castor bean farming provides a vital source of income for small-scale farmers and their families. Castor oil with an ethical source usually originates from vendors that guarantee these farmers decent pay and secure working circumstances. This fairtrade approach helps to lift communities out of poverty, providing them with the financial stability needed to invest in education, healthcare, and other essential services.

Furthermore, companies that prioritize ethical sourcing often invest in community development projects. These initiatives can include building schools, improving healthcare facilities, and providing training for farmers on sustainable agricultural practices. By choosing castor oil from such companies, consumers indirectly contribute to the development and wellbeing of these communities, fostering economic growth and social progress.

The Traceability of castor oil is another important aspect of ethical sourcing. Traceability ensures that the entire supply chain, from the farm to the final product, is transparent and accountable. This transparency helps to prevent exploitation and ensures that the castor oil is produced under humane and ethical conditions. Consumers who opt for ethically sourced castor oil can have confidence that their purchase supports a system that values human rights and environmental stewardship.

Ethical sourcing also emphasizes the importance of fairtrade certification. Products with fair trade certification have been produced and traded under standards that promote environmental sustainability, economic fairness, and social justice. By adhering to these guidelines, farmers may be guaranteed a fair price for their produce that both pays for sustainable production and gives them a livable income. By choosing fair trade certified castor oil, consumers can support a more equitable and sustainable global trade system.

In addition to fair trade, organic certification is another marker of ethically sourced castor oil. Organic certification guarantees that the castor oil is produced without synthetic chemicals, genetically modified organisms (GMOs), or harmful additives. Organic farming practices enhance soil fertility, reduce pollution, and promote biodiversity. Consumers who choose organic castor oil are not only opting for a healthier product but also supporting farming practices that are better for the environment.

The environmental benefits of ethically sourced castor oil extend to the conservation of water resources. Sustainable farming methods often include water conservation practices such as rainwater harvesting, efficient irrigation systems, and soil moisture management. These practices help to reduce water usage and minimize the impact on local water supplies. Given the increasing global concern over water scarcity, supporting products that prioritize water conservation is an important step toward sustainable consumption.

Ethically sourced castor oil also plays a role in mitigating climate change. Sustainable farming practices can sequester carbon in the soil, reduce greenhouse gas emissions, and enhance the resilience of agricultural systems to climate impacts. By choosing castor oil from suppliers committed to these practices, consumers can contribute to the fight against climate change and support a transition to more sustainable agricultural systems.

Choosing ethically sourced castor oil is a decision that extends beyond personal health benefits. It supports sustainable farming practices that protect the environment, promotes fair trade that improves the livelihoods of farmers and contributes to community development. By opting for castor oil from ethical sources, consumers can make a positive impact on local communities and the planet, fostering a more sustainable and equitable global economy. This mindful choice not only ensures the quality and integrity of the product but also aligns with the values of social responsibility and environmental stewardship.

The Impact of Your Choices on the Environment and Global Health

Choosing sustainably produced castor oil has a significant impact on both global health and environmental sustainability. This decision influences a wide range of factors, from the health and wellbeing of farming communities to the preservation of ecosystems and the reduction of greenhouse gas emissions. Choosing castor oil that is produced responsibly encourages agricultural methods that put environmental health first. Synthetic fertilizers and pesticides, which can harm soil quality, taint water supplies, and decrease biodiversity, are frequently used extensively in conventional farming practices. In contrast, sustainable agriculture employs organic fertilizers, crop rotation, and natural pest control methods that maintain soil fertility, reduce pollution, and protect ecosystems.

By choosing castor oil from sustainable sources, consumers support practices that enhance soil health and structure. Healthy soil is more resilient to erosion and can better retain water, reducing the need for irrigation and conserving water resources. Additionally, healthy soil can sequester more carbon, helping to mitigate climate change. The use of organic fertilizers and cover crops further promotes biodiversity, supporting a wide range of plant and animal species.

Water conservation is another crucial benefit of sustainable farming. Conventional farming often requires large amounts of water for irrigation, which can deplete local water supplies and harm aquatic ecosystems. Water consumption is optimized, and waste is decreased by using sustainable farming practices such as rainwater collecting and drip irrigation. This conservation of water resources is essential in regions facing water scarcity and helps to ensure that water remains available for other agricultural and community needs.

Moreover, sustainable castor oil production can reduce greenhouse gas emissions. Carbon dioxide is taken up from the atmosphere and stored in the soil and plants via methods like no till farming, agroforestry, and the use of cover crops. This carbon sequestration is a vital component of climate change mitigation efforts. By supporting sustainably produced castor oil, consumers can contribute to these climate friendly practices and help reduce the overall carbon footprint of agriculture.

The impact of sustainably produced castor oil on global health is multifaceted, affecting both the health of farming communities and the quality of the oil itself. In many developing countries, castor bean farming is a significant source of income for small-scale farmers. Sustainable farming practices often come with certifications like Fair Trade, which ensure that farmers receive fair wages and work in safe conditions. Farmers' general quality of life is raised by their capacity to invest in healthcare, education, and other necessities due to the economy's stability.

Fairtrade and ethical sourcing practices also mean that the working conditions for those involved in castor oil production are safe and humane. This reduces the risk of work-related injuries and illnesses, which are common in agriculture due to exposure to harmful chemicals and unsafe working environments. By choosing castor oil from fair trade sources, consumers support better health and safety standards for workers.

Furthermore, sustainable farming practices reduce the exposure of farming communities to harmful chemicals. The use of synthetic fertilizers and pesticides in traditional farming can result in a variety of health concerns, such as long-term chronic diseases, skin ailments, and respiratory difficulties. Organic farming methods eliminate the use of these harmful substances, creating a healthier environment for farmers and their families.

The benefits of sustainably produced castor oil extend to consumers as well. Organic and sustainably produced castor oil is free from synthetic chemicals and additives, making it a safer and healthier choice for personal use. This is particularly important for products used in personal care and health, where the purity and safety of the ingredients are paramount. By choosing high-quality, sustainably produced castor oil, consumers can minimize the risk of adverse reactions and long-term health effects.

Sustainably produced castor oil also contributes to the economic and social development of farming communities. Fairtrade practices ensure that farmers receive a fair price for their crops, which helps to lift them out of poverty and provides financial stability. This economic empowerment allows farmers to invest in their communities, improving infrastructure, education, and healthcare.

Many companies that prioritize sustainable and ethical sourcing also invest in community development projects. These initiatives can include building schools, improving healthcare facilities, and providing training for farmers on sustainable agricultural practices. By choosing castor oil from such companies, consumers indirectly support these development efforts, fostering economic growth and social progress in producing communities.

The choices consumers make have a powerful influence on market trends and corporate practices. By demanding sustainably produced and ethically sourced castor oil, consumers drive companies to adopt more responsible practices. This market influence can lead to broader systemic changes, encouraging more sustainable and ethical production methods across the industry.

Education and consumer awareness are essential elements of this process. Understanding the environmental and social impacts of conventional versus sustainable farming practices empowers consumers to make informed choices. Certifications such as Fair Trade, Organic, and Rainforest Alliance can guide consumers toward products that meet high standards of sustainability and ethics. Encouraging companies who are open about their sourcing and manufacturing methods guarantee that the things that customers buy reflect their beliefs.

Choosing sustainably produced castor oil has far reaching benefits for both environmental sustainability and global health. It supports farming practices that protect soil health, conserve water, and reduce greenhouse gas emissions, contributing to the fight against climate change. It also promotes fair wages, safe working conditions, and economic stability for farming communities, improving their overall quality of life. For consumers, sustainably produced castor oil offers a safer and healthier product free from harmful chemicals. Customers may influence positive change and promote a more just and sustainable global economy by making educated decisions and supporting moral and sustainable business practices.

CONCLUSION

Bonus Materials

Bonus 1: Checklist to Types of Castor Oil

Choosing the right type of castor oil is essential to ensure you get the most benefits for your specific needs Here is a comprehensive checklist to help you identify and select the best type of castor oil for various applications:

Cold Pressed Castor Oil

Description: Extracted by pressing castor beans without heat, preserving the oil's natural properties.

Best For: Skin and hair care, medicinal uses, and cosmetics.

Benefits: Retains maximum nutrients, high in ricinoleic acid, and free from harmful chemicals.

Organic Castor Oil

Description: Produced from organically grown castor beans without synthetic pesticides or fertilizers.

Best For: Sensitive skin, ecofriendly applications, and internal use

Benefits: Free from harmful chemicals, environmentally friendly, and safer for sensitive skin.

Refined Castor Oil

Description: Processed to remove impurities, resulting in a clear, odorless oil.

Best For: Industrial applications, cosmetics, and some medicinal uses.

Benefits: Longer shelf life, consistent quality, and less odor.

Jamaican Black Castor Oil

Description: Extracted from roasted castor beans, giving it a dark color and a distinct smell.

Best For: Hair growth, scalp treatments, and thickening hair.

Benefits: Rich in ash content from the roasting process, which is believed to have added benefits for hair and scalp health.

Hydrogenated Castor Oil (Castor Wax)

Description: Castor oil that has been hydrogenated to create a solid wax.

Best For: Cosmetics, polishes, and coatings.

Benefits: Solid at room temperature, provides a thickening effect, and is used in various industrial applications.

Pale Pressed Castor Oil

Description: A high-quality oil obtained from the first pressing of castor beans.

Best For: Pharmaceuticals, high-quality cosmetics, and medicinal uses.

Benefits: High purity, minimal impurities, and superior quality.

Dehydrated Castor Oil

Description: Castor oil that has been chemically dehydrated to remove water molecules.

Best For: Paints, coatings, and inks.

Benefits: Provides a nondrying, flexible film, and enhances product durability.

Sulfated Castor Oil (Turkey Red Oil)

Description: Castor oil that has been treated with sulfuric acid to make it water soluble.

Best For: Bath products, emulsifiers, and lubricants.

Benefits: Easily mixes with water, useful in formulations requiring emulsification.

Pharmaceutical Grade Castor Oil

Description: Highly refined castor oil that meets stringent purity standards for medicinal use.

Best For: Laxatives, topical treatments, and pharmaceutical formulations.

Benefits: High purity, safe for internal and medicinal use, and free from contaminants.

Cold Processed Castor Oil

Description: Similar to cold pressed but processed at lower temperatures to retain even more nutrients.

Best For: Skincare, therapeutic uses, and health supplements.

Benefits: Maximizes nutrient retention, gentle on skin, and potent therapeutic properties.

Tips for Choosing the Right Type:

Determine your primary use (e.g, skin care, hair care, industrial, medicinal).

Check for certifications like organic, fair trade, or pharmaceutical grade.

Consider the extraction method to ensure maximum nutrient retention.

Evaluate the purity and presence of additives or chemicals.

Look for reputable brands with transparent sourcing and processing practices.

By using this checklist, you can make informed decisions and select the best type of castor oil to meet your specific needs and preferences.

Bonus 2: Top Brands for Quality Castor Oil

When selecting castor oil, choosing reputable brands ensures you receive a high-quality product that is pure, effective, and ethically sourced Here is a list of top brands known for their quality castor oil products:

1 Sky Organics

Product: Organic Castor Oil.

Highlights: USDA Organic certified, cold pressed, and free from additives Known for its high purity and nutrient retention.

Best For: Skin care, hair care, and general health applications.

2 Heritage Store

Product: Castor Oil

Highlights: Cold pressed, hexane free, and free from synthetic chemicals Available in both regular and organic versions.

Best For: Skin and hair treatments, massages, and medicinal uses.

3 Now Solutions

Product: Castor Oil.

Highlights: Cold pressed, hexane free, and pure Known for its consistent quality and affordability.

Best For: Moisturizing skin, conditioning hair, and therapeutic applications.

4 Kate Blanc Cosmetics

Product: Organic Castor Oil.

Highlights: USDA Organic certified, cold pressed, and pure Packaged with a glass dropper for easy application.

Best For: Enhancing hair growth, nourishing skin, and strengthening nails.

5 Molivera Organics

Product: Castor Oil.

Highlights: Cold pressed, unrefined, and free from hexane Highly rated for its effectiveness and purity.

Best For: Hair and scalp treatments, skin hydration, and eyebrow and eyelash growth.

6 Aria Starr

Product: Castor Oil.

Highlights: Cold pressed, unrefined, and pure Comes with a pump dispenser for convenience.

Best For: Deep conditioning hair, treating dry skin, and promoting hair growth.

7 Majestic Pure

Product: Castor Oil.

Highlights: Cold pressed, hexane free, and pure Known for its high quality and multipurpose use.

Best For: Skin care, hair care, and natural remedies.

8 Handcraft Blends

Product: 00% Pure Castor Oil.

Highlights: Cold pressed, hexane free, and unrefined Comes in a dark amber bottle to protect from UV rays.

Best For: Hair and scalp health, moisturizing skin, and therapeutic uses.

9 Organic Castor Oil by Eve Hansen

Product: Organic Castor Oil.

Highlights: USDA Organic certified, cold pressed, and pure Packaged in a glass bottle with a dropper for easy application.

Best For: Boosting hair growth, skin nourishment, and DIY beauty treatments.

10 Tropic Isle Living

Product: Jamaican Black Castor Oil.

Highlights: Authentic Jamaican black castor oil, roasted and cold pressed Known for its rich nutrient content and traditional processing.

Best For: Thickening hair, treating scalp issues, and enhancing hair growth.

Tips for Choosing Quality Castor Oil:

Look for Cold Pressed: Cold pressed castor oil retains more nutrients and beneficial properties compared to heat extracted oils.

Check for Organic Certification: USDA Organic certified oils ensure that the product is free from synthetic pesticides and fertilizers.

Verify Purity: Pure castor oil should be free from hexane, additives, and synthetic ingredients.

Read Reviews: Customer reviews and ratings can provide insights into the effectiveness and quality of the product.

 Packaging: Dark glass bottles protect the oil from light exposure, preserving its quality and extending its shelf life.

By choosing from these top brands, you can be confident in the quality and effectiveness of the castor oil you purchase, ensuring the best results for your health and beauty needs.

Bonus 3: Castor Oil Myths and Misconceptions

Castor oil has been used for centuries in various cultures for its numerous health benefits However, along with its popularity, several myths and misconceptions have emerged Understanding these myths and the truths behind them can help you make informed decisions about using castor oil effectively and safely.

Myth 1: Castor Oil is Toxic

Misconception: Some people believe that castor oil is toxic and unsafe for use.

Truth: Castor oil is derived from the seeds of the castor plant (Ricinus communis), which contain ricin, a highly toxic substance However, the extraction process for castor oil removes ricin, making the oil safe for topical and internal use Pharmaceutical-grade and food-grade castor oil are extensively purified and are safe when used as directed.

Myth 2: Castor Oil Causes Hair to Grow Overnight

Misconception: Many believe that applying castor oil will result in immediate hair growth.

Truth: While castor oil is beneficial for hair health and can promote hair growth over time, it does not produce instant results Consistent use over several weeks or months is necessary to see noticeable improvements in hair thickness and length Castor oil works by nourishing the scalp, improving blood circulation, and strengthening hair follicles.

Myth 3: Castor Oil Should Only Be Used Externally

Misconception: Some people think castor oil is only for external use and is unsafe for internal consumption.

Truth: Castor oil is safe for internal use when consumed in appropriate amounts It has been traditionally used as a natural laxative to relieve constipation However, it is essential to follow recommended dosages and consult with a healthcare provider before using castor oil internally, especially for individuals with underlying health conditions.

Myth 4: Castor Oil is Not Suitable for Sensitive Skin

Misconception: There is a belief that castor oil can cause irritation and should not be used on sensitive skin.

Truth: Castor oil is generally well-tolerated and has anti-inflammatory properties that can benefit sensitive skin However, as with any new product, it is advisable to perform a patch test before widespread use This helps ensure that the individual does not have an allergic reaction or sensitivity to the oil.

Myth 5: All Castor Oils are the Same

Misconception: Some people assume that all castor oil products are identical in quality and effectiveness.

Truth: The quality of castor oil can vary significantly depending on the extraction method, source, and processing Cold pressed, organic, and hexane free castor oils are generally of higher quality and retain more beneficial properties It is important to choose castor oil from reputable brands that follow stringent quality standards.

Myth 6: Castor Oil Can Cure Serious Diseases

Misconception: Some claims suggest that castor oil can cure serious diseases such as cancer.

Truth: While castor oil has many health benefits, it is not a cure for serious diseases Its primary uses include skin and hair care, relief from constipation, and minor pain management. For serious medical conditions, it is crucial to seek appropriate medical treatment and not rely solely on natural remedies like castor oil.

Myth 7: Castor Oil Can Be Used in Large Quantities Safely

Misconception: There is a belief that using more castor oil will enhance its benefits.

Truth: Using excessive amounts of castor oil, especially internally, can lead to adverse effects such as diarrhea, cramping, and dehydration It is important to follow recommended dosages and application guidelines to avoid negative side effects More is not always better when it comes to using castor oil.

Myth 8: Castor Oil Only Benefits Hair Growth

Misconception: Some people think castor oil is only effective for promoting hair growth

Truth: Castor oil has a wide range of uses beyond hair growth It is beneficial for moisturizing skin, reducing inflammation, relieving minor pain, and treating conditions like dandruff and dry scalp Its versatile properties make it a valuable addition to various beauty and health routines.

Myth 9: Castor Oil Should Be Heated Before Use

Misconception: It is commonly believed that castor oil must be heated to be effective.

Truth: While warming castor oil slightly can enhance its absorption and soothing properties, it is not necessary for its effectiveness Castor oil can be used at room temperature for most applications, and it retains its beneficial properties without heating.

Myth 10: Castor Oil Works the Same for Everyone

Misconception: There is a belief that castor oil will have the same effects on everyone who uses it.

Truth: The effectiveness of castor oil can vary from person to person due to individual differences in skin type, hair type, and overall health While many people experience positive results, others may not see the same benefits It is important to set realistic expectations and understand that results may vary.

Understanding these myths and misconceptions about castor oil helps in making informed decisions and using this versatile oil safely and effectively. By choosing high-quality products and following appropriate usage guidelines, you can maximize the benefits of castor oil for your health and beauty needs.

You've Reached the End!

Thank you for reading our book to the end We hope you've found it helpful and informative Your opinion matters greatly to us.

Why Your Review Matters:

Your review helps us improve and lets other readers know what to expect from this book Sharing your experience can make a significant impact

How You Can Share Your Review:

- Through Amazon.com:
- Go to the Amazon page where you found my book.
- Navigate to the 'Customer Reviews' section.

Click on 'Write a customer review' to share your valuable insights.

Instant QR Code Access: Simply scan the QR code below with your smartphone to be directed to the Amazon review section.

We appreciate your time and support!